A Handbook for DEALING WITH SUGAR CRAVINGS and Dependency

NCWC's Nutrition 101 Series

A. Sehatti, RN, MSN
Family Nurse Practitioner

NCWC/Amend-Health Press

A HANDBOOK FOR DEALING WITH SUGAR CRAVINGS AND DEPENDENCY. NCWC'S NUTRITION 101 SERIES. Copyright © 2021 by A. Sehatti, RN, MSN, Family Nurse Practitioner.

All rights reserved.

No part of this book may be reproduced in whole or in part, translated, stored in a retrieval system, or transmitted, in any form or by any means such as recording, electronic, mechanical, microfilming, or otherwise, without the prior written permission of the author (A. Sehatti, RN, MSN, FNP) or Amend-Health Press.

ISBN 978-0-578-88723-4 (paperback)

1. Diabetes   2. Insulin Resistance   3. Dependency/Addiction   4. Lifestyle Changes
5. Weight Loss   I. Title   II. A. Sehatti

Printed and bounded in the United States of America
First Printing Copyrighted: March 2021
Revised Editions Copyrighted: May 2021, November 2021, November 2022

Published by:
NCWC/Amend-Health Press
AKA Nutritional Counseling and Weight Control Clinic
51 E. Campbell Avenue, Suite 129 - 154
Campbell, CA 95008
United States
www.NCWC-AmendHealthPress.com
www.EatActThinkHealthy.com

About the Author

A. Sehatti is a registered nurse and family nurse practitioner. She received her bachelor's degree in nursing from University of Pennsylvania and her master's degree in nursing from UCLA.

Aside from her clinical work at such places as Stanford, UCLA, and Caltech Health Center, Ms. Sehatti has over forty years of experience in educating adults and children on total wellness. She currently works as a health educator and nutritional consultant at a private practice that she established in 2005 in Northern California.

A. Sehatti is highly dedicated to making a difference in people's lives. It has been the reward of witnessing people reach their health and wellness goals that has inspired her to write books and share the tools that have helped her clients with her readers.

Books Published by A. Sehatti

A TOOL FOR LETTING GO OF RESENTMENT AND ANGER
Short. Straightforward. Transformative.

ACCOUNTABILITY AND EMPOWERMENT
A Four-Step Strategy for Overcoming Resentment

BUILDING A STRONG SENSE OF SELF
Embarking on the Journey of Change

THE INNER CONTROL IS THE TRUE CONTROL WORKBOOK, SECOND EDITION
Inspirational Scripts

A WORKBOOK FOR OVERCOMING RESENTMENT
Mindfulness Scripts

NCWC'S NUTRITION 101 WORKBOOK
NCWC's Nutrition 101 Series

21-DAY LOG BOOK FOR ACHIEVING WELLNESS GOALS
NCWC's Nutrition 101 Series

Contents

Added Sugar

Added sugar refers to the sugar(s) that we or manufacturers add to the foods that we eat in order to improve their taste or extend their shelf life (see Page 8).

So, is eating a lot of added sugar really bad for us? Let's explore some of the health effects of high sugar consumption and then decide for ourselves.

Inflammation: Eating too much added sugar on a regular basis can cause chronic inflammation in our body.

Inflammation can be a normal response by our immune system when our body is faced with a physiological stressor, such as an injury, infection, emotional trauma, or exposure to a substance that appears harmful or foreign to the body.

Chronic inflammation happens when this inflammatory response lingers on and becomes persistent and ongoing.

A chronic low-grade inflammation can lead to such health problems as:

Cardiovascular Disorders: Chronic inflammation in the walls of our arteries can cause scarring. This can narrow or block our blood vessels and lead to such diseases as high blood pressure, heart attack, and stroke.

Additionally, elevated levels of C-Reactive Protein, which is a marker for inflammation, has been associated with increased levels of LDL (the bad cholesterol). High levels of LDL that build up on the wall of our arteries can lead to blood clots, heart disease, and other cardiovascular diseases.

Cancer: Studies have shown that chronic inflammation can damage our cells (i.e., our DNA) and puts us at a greater risk for developing cancer.

Gastrointestinal (GI) disorders: Inflammation in the lining of our digestive tract can lead to such GI problems as inflammatory bowel disease (IBS) and Crohn's disease flare-ups. Studies have also linked chronic inflammation to non-alcoholic fatty liver disease.

Weight gains: Inflammation in the GI tract also increases the growth of bad bacteria in our gut. An imbalance in our gut bacteria (having less good bacteria than the bad) can lead to weight gains.

Joint problems: Worsening joint pains and a higher risk of developing rheumatoid arthritis have been linked to the chronic inflammation caused by high amounts of added-sugar in our diet.

Aging of the skin: The excess amounts of sugar that we consume binds with many different proteins in our blood-stream and forms compounds that damage the collagen in our skin.

Endocrine Problems: When we keep eating foods that have high amounts of sugar, our pancreas, which secretes insulin to keep our blood sugar levels normal, becomes overtaxed. An overworked pancreas can lead to high blood sugar levels, type 2 diabetes, and insulin resistance.

When the cells in our body become resistant to insulin, we end up having higher levels of sugar in our bloodstream.

As our blood sugar rises, our pancreas pumps out more and more insulin. The excess insulin stimulates the ovaries to produce more androgens. An overproduction of androgens is associated with polycystic ovary syndrome (PCOS). This may explain why controlling sugar consumption can significantly improve PCOS.

Dopamine Effect: Eating sweets and foods that have high amounts of added sugar stimulates the reward center of our brain and triggers the release of dopamine, a chemical that makes us experience pleasure.

Just like other substances that stimulate the release of dopamine (i.e., alcohol), our brain develops tolerance: we need more and more sugar to have the same experience and feel good. This may explain why we crave and become sugar dependent over time.

Studies have linked high intake of added sugar to imbalances in the levels of dopamine and other chemicals in our brain and concluded that these imbalances can put us at risk for developing mood swings and depression.

For the most part, we don't have to deprive ourselves of the foods that we love.

We can maintain our control without taking away pleasure in life.

We can achieve this goal by practicing moderation and setting limits:

How much and how often we have foods that are high in added sugar.

Studies have shown that eating too much refined carbohydrates (i.e., white rice, pasta, foods made with white flour, and many cereals) can also lead to inflammation, endocrine problems, and dopamine imbalance.

About This Book

A Handbook for Dealing With Sugar Cravings and Dependency outlines a set of dietary, physical activity, and behavioral strategies for managing sugar cravings. These helpful tips are simple, practical, easy to follow, and straightforward.

Additionally, this book raises your awareness, triggers thoughts, and encourages you to look at the emotional factors that may contribute to your cravings—an important step in maintaining healthy lifestyle changes.

This handbook also provides you with a tool that will help you gradually reduce your sugar intake over the course of eight weeks and achieve your health goals.

A Handbook for Dealing With Sugar Cravings and Dependency is designed according to the nutrition education curriculum offered by A. Sehatti, RN, MSN, FNP at NCWC (Nutritional Counseling and Weight Control Clinic).

Please note that the knowledge shared in this book can change over time based on the latest scientific findings that are discovered. Moreover, the information provided by the author is not intended to be complete or exhaustive nor is it a substitute for the advice and/or prescription offered to you by your primary care provider.

For more information, references, and review of research studies on added sugar consumption and its health impacts, refer to such sources and publications as American Diabetes Association, American Heart Association, Mayo Clinic, Harvard Health, Cleveland Health, and John Hopkins Medicine.

1

Goals

1. Lose sugar / sweet taste

2. Limit maximum daily added sugar consumption:

   Women: About 6 teaspoons = 100 calories
   Men: About 9 teaspoons = 150 calories

   Source: American Heart Association

Dietary Measures to Control Sugar Cravings

Gain Knowledge, Set Realistic Goals,
Make Plans, and Commit.

A. Take baby steps and gradually reduce the added sugar in your diet (i.e., in your coffee, tea, or cereal).

B. Avoid artificial sweeteners.

C. Limit consumption of honey or brown sugar which may be perceived as healthy sugars.

D. Limit processed foods which hide loads of sugar.

E. Maintain a steady blood sugar during the day:

   » Avoid hunger;
   » Eat three well-balanced meals; and,
   » Include healthy snacks at mid-morning and mid-afternoon.

F. Include raw vegetables in your daily diet.

G. Eat *fresh* fruits (2 to 3 servings per day).

H. Read labels and avoid foods that include High Fructose Corn Syrup in their ingredients.

I. Avoid/limit regular or diet soft drinks.

J. Drink water. (Please note that drinking too much water can result in serious health consequences.)

K. Avoid/limit cocktail mixes (use sensible amounts of fresh squeezed fruit juice instead).

L. Read the ingredient listings carefully:

   » A food may be high in added sugar when any form of it (Page 8) appears as one of the first three ingredients on the list.

   » A food may also be high in added sugar when several forms of sugar appear on its product's ingredient list.

   » Look for hidden sugar in such items as:

      ◦ Salad dressings (particularly, reduced-fat ones)
      ◦ Flavored coffee or tea drinks
      ◦ Baked beans
      ◦ Bread
      ◦ BBQ sauce
      ◦ Pasta sauce
      ◦ Ketchup
      ◦ _______________________________________
      ◦ _______________________________________
      ◦ _______________________________________
      ◦ _______________________________________
      ◦ _______________________________________
      ◦ _______________________________________
      ◦ _______________________________________
      ◦ _______________________________________
      ◦ _______________________________________
      ◦ _______________________________________

M. The followings are used in ingredient listings to describe the different forms of sugar / sweeteners that are added to foods:

Sucrose	Corn syrup
Fructose	Corn sweetener
Maltose	Fruit juice concentrate
Lactose	Agave nectar
Dextrose	Evaporated cane juice
Glucose	Cane juice
Honey	Barbados sugar
Molasses	Barley malt
Syrup	Barley malt syrup
Brown rice syrup	Beet sugar
Brown sugar	Buttered syrup
Malt syrup	High-fructose corn syrup
Maple syrup	Ethyl Maltol

N. For curbing cravings, include healthy snacks that have fiber and protein. The followings are some examples of such snacks:

<table>
<tr><td>

Fruit (one serving) + Dairy (one serving)

(i.e., 1 fresh apple with the skin + 6 oz plain Greek yogurt)

</td></tr>
<tr><td>

Fresh fruit (one serving) + Nut (one serving)

(i.e., 1 fresh orange + 1/4 cup unsalted almonds)

</td></tr>
<tr><td>

Raw veggies (1-2 serving) + Nut (one servings)

(i.e., 1 cup raw baby carrots + 1/4 cup unsalted almonds)

</td></tr>
<tr><td>

Raw veggies (1-2 serving) + Dairy (one servings)

(i.e., 1 cup raw baby carrots + 6 oz plain Greek yogurt)

</td></tr>
<tr><td>

Fresh fruit (one serving) + Raw veggies (one servings)

(i.e., 1 fresh orange + 1 small raw bell pepper)

</td></tr>
</table>

O. Limit/Avoid MSG (Monosodium Glutamate).

P. Read ingredients carefully. If the food contains such ingredients as one of the followings then it may contain MSG:

Seasoning
Spices
Enzymes
Flavoring (i.e., Natural flavoring or Malt flavoring)
Yeast extract, food, or nutrient
Glutamate
Caseinate
Hydrolyzed
Amino acid
Malt extract
Bouillon
Broth stock or Natural beef/chicken flavor
Vegetable protein
Protein-fortified
Autolyzed plant protein
Soy protein isolate or concentrate
Whey protein isolate or concentrate

Adopted from US Food & Drug Administration (FDA)

Physical Activity Tips for Dealing With Sugar Cravings

*Set a Goal, Make Plans, and Be Active
While Having Fun.*

A. Engage in daily aerobic exercises / cardio workouts (cardiovascular conditioning):

>   » *Definition*: Any moderate-paced activity, sustained for at least 10 minutes, that increases our breathing and heart rate through continuous, repetitive, and rhythmic movement of the large muscle groups of arms and legs may be considered as an aerobic exercise.

>   » *Examples*: Brisk walking, swimming, dancing, and jogging

>   » *Duration*: At least 30 minutes

B. Include weight bearing exercises:

>   » *Definition*: Any activity in which the repeated contractions of the major muscle groups (i.e., our abdomen, arms, legs, and chest) against a weight or force (i.e., our own body weight, free weights, weight machines, or exercise bands) are sustained for about 10 seconds or more can be considered as a muscle strengthening activity. (Lower intensity and higher repetition is recommended.)

>   » *Examples*: Push-ups and sit-ups; pilates; yoga workouts; working out using dumbbells, bands, or weight machines

>   » *Duration*: One or more sets of 12 repetitions of such exercises performed three times per week

C. Avoid/Limit sedentary activities:

>> *Definition*: A Sedentary activity may be defined as any activity that we engage in for an average of 8 hours or more per day that doesn't increase the body's energy expenditure much above the resting level.

>> *Examples*: Lying down; sitting; watching television; working/reading/playing on a computer or cell phone; playing video games

D. Some helpful tips:

>> Track your daily steps

>> Set limits for such sedentary activities as watching TV or playing electronic games

>> Set reminders (i.e., on your phone) to take short breaks for getting up and moving around when you have to sit at a desk

>> Commit to your physical activity goal by making realistic and achievable plans

>> Adjust your goal/plans when circumstances change (i.e., be flexible and overcome *all-or-nothing* way of thinking)

>> To turn your physical activity into a daily routine, keep a daily log and aim for progression, not perfection

Please consult your healthcare professional before starting a new exercise program or workout routine, especially if you are diagnosed with such chronic health problems as hypertension, heart disease, diabetes, cancer, or arthritis.

Behavior Modification Strategies for Managing Sugar Cravings

Acknowledge, Gain Awareness, and Become Proactive.

A. Be true to yourself.

B. Acknowledge the problem.

C. Have a realistic outlook:

> » This may be a lifelong process.
> » Relapses are natural parts of this process.

D. Gain insight into yourself:

> » Become aware of your self-talks;
> » Know what triggers your sugar cravings; and,
> » Make a list of these trigger factors (i.e., boredom, hunger, anxiety, stress):

> > o _______________________________________
> >
> > o _______________________________________
> >
> > o _______________________________________
> >
> > o _______________________________________
> >
> > o _______________________________________
> >
> > o _______________________________________
> >
> > o _______________________________________
> >
> > o _______________________________________
> >
> > o _______________________________________
> >
> > o _______________________________________

E. Identify other cravings and/or dependencies that you may be experiencing, such as salt cravings (i.e., craving for hummus or salted nuts):

» _______________________________________

» _______________________________________

» _______________________________________

» _______________________________________

» _______________________________________

» _______________________________________

» _______________________________________

» _______________________________________

» _______________________________________

F. Become aware of your unhealthy relationship patterns which trigger such self-soothing behaviors as turning to sweets for comfort (Avoidance Coping):

» Keep a journal;
» Record your self-discoveries; and,
» List the unhealthy dynamics in your relationships that trigger sugar cravings:

» _______________________________________

» _______________________________________

» _______________________________________

» _______________________________________

» _______________________________________

» _______________________________________

» _______________________________________

» _______________________________________

» _______________________________________

G. Cultivate mindfulness by exploring such concepts as:

> » Moderation vs. rigidity (i.e., portion control vs. self-deprivation)
> » Self-compassion vs. self-indulgence
> » Actions vs. reactions (i.e., rational choices vs. rationalizations)
> » Regret vs. remorse (i.e., self-accountability vs. self-depreciation)

H. For gaining more awareness refer to *Building A Strong Sense of Self: Embarking on the Journey of Change.*

I. For exploring and cultivating healthy coping behaviors refer to *Accountability and Empowerment: A Four-Step Strategy for Overcoming Resentment.*

*"Just as a tree, though cut down, can grow again
and again if its roots are undamaged and strong,
in the same way if the roots of craving are not wholly
uprooted, sorrows will come again and again."*
—Gautama Buddha

Preventing and Managing Setbacks

A. Commit to realistic goals (i.e., take baby steps) and make feasible and sustainable plans to reach them.

B. Recognize, identify, and make a list of all the signs and symptoms of sugar withdrawal that you experience when you reduce your sugar consumption. Some examples of such signs/symptoms may be:

- » Cravings
- » Headaches
- » Irritability
- » Fatigue
- » Cognitive problems
- » Restlessness
- » Anxiety

- » ____
- » ____
- » ____
- » ____
- » ____
- » ____
- » ____

C. Anticipate these signs or symptoms before they happen and have a plan to deal with them. For example, plan to:
- » Use the STOP SIGN: Stop. Think. Act.
- » Eat a healthy snack that contains fiber and protein (Page 9).
- » Go for a 30-minute brisk walk.

D. Implement your plan at the onset, before full withdrawal signs or symptoms appear.

E. Learn from setbacks through self-reflection.

F. Cultivate a constructive mindset (refer to *The Inner Control is the True Control Workbook, 2nd Edition*):

View relapses or regressions to old habits as a learning opportunity and a stepping stone to success.

*"It is only by going down into the abyss
that we recover the treasures of life.
Where you stumble, there lies your treasure."*
—Joseph Campbell

Other Behavioral Changes

A. Change your eating habits:

   » Eat whole, natural/real, and fresh foods.
   » Limit or avoid packaged, bottled, or canned foods.
   » Eat foods with five or less ingredients.
   » Eat out or take in less often.
   » Keep daily food logs (refer to *21-Day Log Book for Achieving Wellness Goals*).

B. Remove tempting foods that have loads of sugar from your immediate environment (i.e., pantry or workplace).

C. Clean out your pantry and fridge to reduce the temptation to bake or cook unhealthy foods.

D. Other measures:

____

____

____

____

____

____

____

____

____

____

____

____

____

2
Intervention

1. Identify and list all the sources of added sugar in your current daily diet, such as in your coffee/tea drinks, other beverages, and cocktails; sauces and salad dressings; bread, cereal, baked beans, and snacks (Page 22).

2. Record the amount of calories these food items generally contribute to your daily/weekly calorie intake (Page 22).

3. Establish a baseline: Reflect on the past week and try to recall the number of times that you experienced cravings; the number of times that you gave in to your temptations; and, the number of calories that you consumed to satisfy those cravings / temptations over the course of that week (Page 24).

4. Work towards reducing added sugar in your diet every week:

   a. Set a realistic goal and make concrete plans for the upcoming week (Page 25).

   "A goal without a plan is just a wish."
   —Antoine de Saint-Exupéry

   b. Aim for progression, not perfection.

5. Record all deviations from your daily plans (i.e., the instances that you didn't follow through with the plans that you had made because you *struggled to overcome your temptations* or because you *mindlessly made a poor choice*) (Page 27).

6. Find out the amount of calories those deviations from your plans contributed to your *daily* calorie intake (Page 27).

7. Evaluate your progress by recording:

    a. The number of times you experienced cravings over the week that has passed;
    b. The number of times you deviated from your original plans; and,
    c. The number of calories those deviations added to your total calorie intake for that *week* (Page 28).

8. Make time for self-reflection: Work through *the Genuine Accountability Process* and hold yourself accountable for the negatives outcomes without being self-critical (refer to *Accountability and Empowerment*) (Page 29):

    a. Understand what happened;
    b. Learn from mistakes;
    c. Adjust your goal;
    d. Make new and more sustainable plans; and,
    e. Commit to your new learnings.

9. Create an incentive program: Without using food, reward yourself when you reach your weekly goal.

10. Repeat Steps 4 through 9 for the next seven weeks (Page 31).

11. Review the dietary, activity, and behavioral tips that are offered in this handbook *regularly* and as needed.

12. After completing this eight-week program, retake Steps 1 through 11 as soon as you notice that the old habits are coming back.

Summary: The Steps of the Intervention Process
1. Identify the sources of added sugar in your *current* daily diet and record the amount of calories these food items contribute to your daily calorie intake (Page 22)
2. Establish a baseline (Page 24)
3. Set a realistic goal and make concrete plans to reduce added sugar in your diet for the upcoming week (Page 25)
4. Record all deviations from your daily plans and the amount of calories these deviations add to your daily calorie intake (Page 27)
5. Evaluate your progress (Page 28)
6. Hold yourself accountable for your mistakes, learn from them, adjust your goals/plans, and commit to your new learnings. (Page 29)
7. Repeat Steps 4 through 9 for the next seven weeks (Page 31)

What Are the Sources of Added Sugar in Your Current Daily Diet?

Food	Calories

Food	Calories
	23

How many times did you experience sugar
cravings over the past 7 days?

____

How many times did you give in to your
temptations/cravings over the past 7 days?

____

How many calories did those foods (that you
consumed to satisfy your cravings) add to your
total calorie intake for the past week?

____

Week 1: Your Goal and Plans for Reducing Added Sugar in Your Daily Diet

Goal(s):	
Day	**Plan(s)**
Monday	
Tuesday	
Wednesday	
Thursday	
Friday	
Saturday	
Sunday	

Comments

Week 1 (Cont'd)

Day	Time	Deviations From Plan(s)	Calories	Comments
Monday				
Tuesday				
Wednesday				
Thursday				
Friday				
Saturday				
Sunday				

Self-Evaluation

How many times did you experience sugar cravings over the past 7 days?

____

How many times did you deviate from your original plans and give in to your temptations/cravings over the past 7 days?

____

How many calories have those deviations from your plans added to your total calorie intake for the past week?

____

Total of 3500 calories = 1 pound of body fat

Self-Reflection

*Hold yourself accountable for the deviation(s) from
your plan(s) without being self-critical.*

A. Understand what happened;
B. Learn from your mistakes;
C. Adjust your goal;
D. Make new and more sustainable plan(s); and,
E. Commit to your new learnings.

> *Self-accountability is not about
> blaming ourselves; Rather, it is about taking
> responsibility for the choices we make.*

> *Self-accountability helps us stay
> in control and see choices, while blaming
> ourselves for our mistakes makes us
> feel frustrated and stuck.*

Week 2: Your Goal and Plans for Reducing Added Sugar in Your Daily Diet

Goal(s):	
Day	**Plan(s)**
Monday	
Tuesday	
Wednesday	
Thursday	
Friday	
Saturday	
Sunday	

Comments

Week 2 (Cont'd)

Day	Time	Deviations From Plan(s)	Calories	Comments
Monday				
Tuesday				
Wednesday				
Thursday				
Friday				
Saturday				
Sunday				

Self-Evaluation

How many times did you experience sugar cravings over the past 7 days?

____

How many times did you deviate from your original plans and give in to your temptations/cravings over the past 7 days?

____

How many calories have those deviations from your plans added to your total calorie intake for the past week?

____

> *Total of 3500 calories = 1 pound of body fat*

Self-Reflection

*Hold yourself accountable for the deviation(s) from
your plan(s) without being self-critical.*

A. Understand what happened;
B. Learn from your mistakes;
C. Adjust your goal;
D. Make new and more sustainable plan(s); and,
E. Commit to your new learnings.

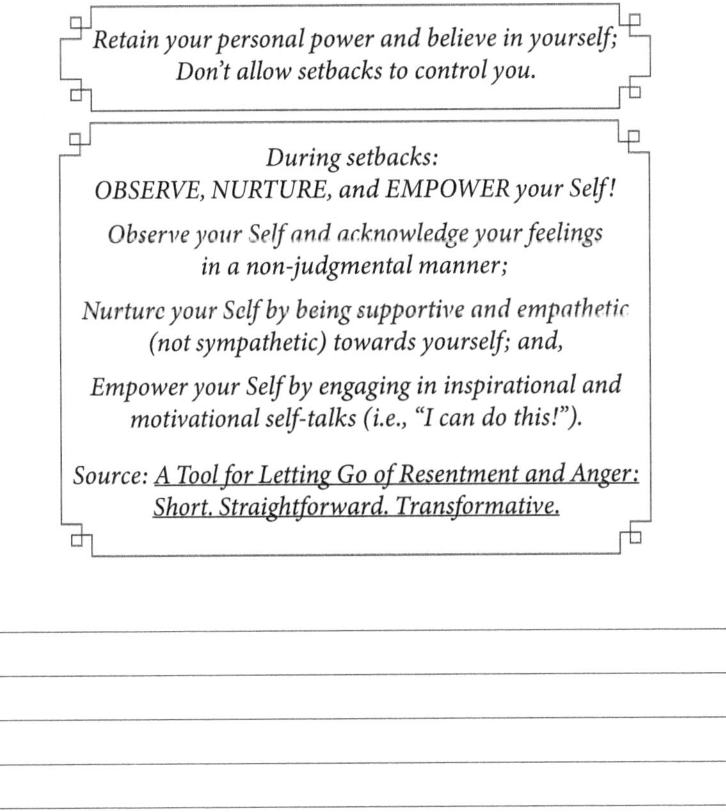

*During setbacks:
OBSERVE, NURTURE, and EMPOWER your Self!*

*Observe your Self and acknowledge your feelings
in a non-judgmental manner;*

*Nurture your Self by being supportive and empathetic
(not sympathetic) towards yourself; and,*

*Empower your Self by engaging in inspirational and
motivational self-talks (i.e., "I can do this!").*

*Source: <u>A Tool for Letting Go of Resentment and Anger:
Short. Straightforward. Transformative.</u>*

Week 3: Your Goal and Plans for Reducing Added Sugar in Your Daily Diet

Day	Plan(s)
Goal(s):	
Monday	
Tuesday	
Wednesday	
Thursday	
Friday	
Saturday	
Sunday	

Comments

Week 3 (Cont'd)

Day	Time	Deviations From Plan(s)	Calories	Comments
Monday				
Tuesday				
Wednesday				
Thursday				
Friday				
Saturday				
Sunday				

Self-Evaluation

How many times did you experience sugar
cravings over the past 7 days?

____

How many times did you deviate from
your original plans and give in to your
temptations/cravings over the past 7 days?

____

How many calories have those deviations
from your plans added to your total
calorie intake for the past week?

____

Total of 3500 calories = 1 pound of body fat

Self-Reflection

*Hold yourself accountable for the deviation(s) from
your plan(s) without being self-critical.*

A. Understand what happened;
B. Learn from your mistakes;
C. Adjust your goal;
D. Make new and more sustainable plan(s); and,
E. Commit to your new learnings.

> *Live your life by aiming
> for progression,
> not perfection.*

Week 4: Your Goal and Plans for Reducing Added Sugar in Your Daily Diet

Goal(s):	
Day	**Plan(s)**
Monday	
Tuesday	
Wednesday	
Thursday	
Friday	
Saturday	
Sunday	

Comments

Week 4 (Cont'd)

Day	Time	Deviations From Plan(s)	Calories	Comments
Monday				
Tuesday				
Wednesday				
Thursday				
Friday				
Saturday				
Sunday				

Self-Evaluation

How many times did you experience sugar cravings over the past 7 days?

____

How many times did you deviate from your original plans and give in to your temptations/cravings over the past 7 days?

____

How many calories have those deviations from your plans added to your total calorie intake for the past week?

____

Total of 3500 calories = 1 pound of body fat

Self-Reflection

*Hold yourself accountable for the deviation(s) from
your plan(s) without being self-critical.*

A. Understand what happened;
B. Learn from your mistakes;
C. Adjust your goal;
D. Make new and more sustainable plan(s); and,
E. Commit to your new learnings.

> *Look at the rear view window only to move onward.*
>
> *Source: <u>A Tool for Letting Go of Resentment and Anger</u>:
> <u>Short. Straightforward. Transformative.</u>*

Week 5: Your Goal and Plans for Reducing Added Sugar in Your Daily Diet

Goal(s):

Day	Plan(s)
Monday	
Tuesday	
Wednesday	
Thursday	
Friday	
Saturday	
Sunday	

Comments

Week 5 (Cont'd)

Day	Time	Deviations From Plan(s)	Calories	Comments
Monday				
Tuesday				
Wednesday				
Thursday				
Friday				
Saturday				
Sunday				

Self-Evaluation

How many times did you experience sugar cravings over the past 7 days?

____

How many times did you deviate from your original plans and give in to your temptations/cravings over the past 7 days?

____

How many calories have those deviations from your plans added to your total calorie intake for the past week?

____

Total of 3500 calories = 1 pound of body fat

Self-Reflection

Hold yourself accountable for the deviation(s) from your plan(s) without being self-critical.

A. Understand what happened;
B. Learn from your mistakes;
C. Adjust your goal;
D. Make new and more sustainable plan(s); and,
E. Commit to your new learnings.

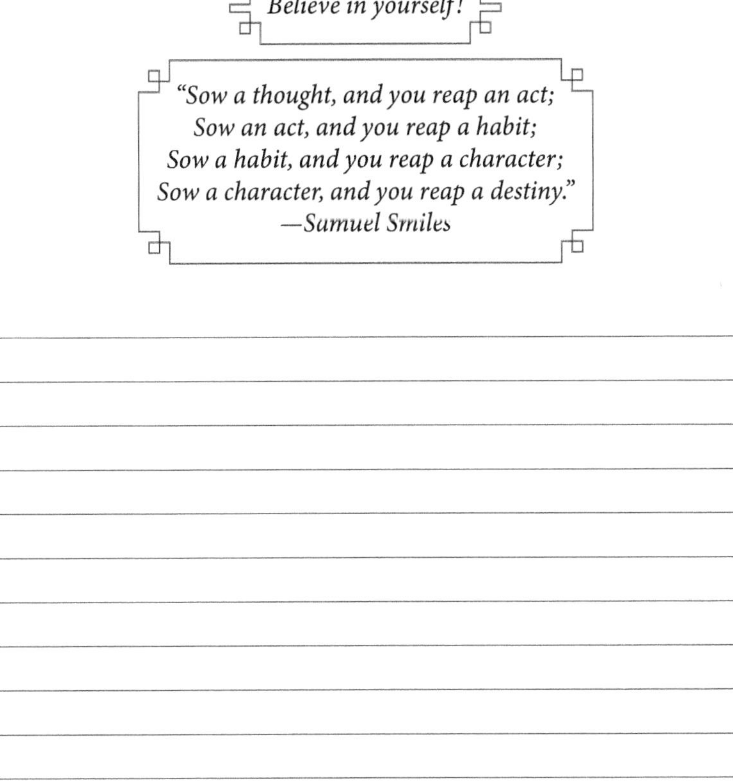

Week 6: Your Goal and Plans for Reducing Added Sugar in Your Daily Diet

Goal(s):	

Day	Plan(s)
Monday	
Tuesday	
Wednesday	
Thursday	
Friday	
Saturday	
Sunday	

Comments

Week 6 (Cont'd)

Day	Time	Deviations From Plan(s)	Calories	Comments
Monday				
Tuesday				
Wednesday				
Thursday				
Friday				
Saturday				
Sunday				

Self-Evaluation

How many times did you experience sugar
cravings over the past 7 days?

____

How many times did you deviate from
your original plans and give in to your
temptations/cravings over the past 7 days?

____

How many calories have those deviations
from your plans added to your total
calorie intake for the past week?

____

Total of 3500 calories = 1 pound of body fat

Self-Reflection

Hold yourself accountable for the deviation(s) from your plan(s) without being self-critical.

A. Understand what happened;
B. Learn from your mistakes;
C. Adjust your goal;
D. Make new and more sustainable plan(s); and,
E. Commit to your new learnings.

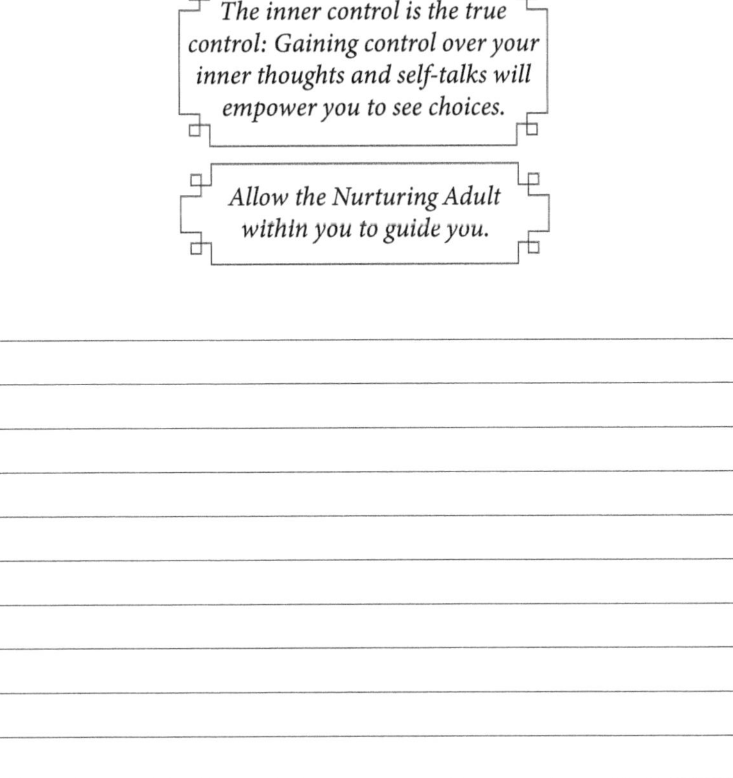

Week 7: Your Goal and Plans for Reducing Added Sugar in Your Daily Diet

Goal(s):	
Day	**Plan(s)**
Monday	
Tuesday	
Wednesday	
Thursday	
Friday	
Saturday	
Sunday	

Comments

Week 7 (Cont'd)

Day	Time	Deviations From Plan(s)	Calories	Comments
Monday				
Tuesday				
Wednesday				
Thursday				
Friday				
Saturday				
Sunday				

Self-Evaluation

How many times did you experience sugar cravings over the past 7 days?

____

How many times did you deviate from your original plans and give in to your temptations/cravings over the past 7 days?

____

How many calories have those deviations from your plans added to your total calorie intake for the past week?

____

Total of 3500 calories = 1 pound of body fat

Self-Reflection

*Hold yourself accountable for the deviation(s) from
your plan(s) without being self-critical.*

A. Understand what happened;
B. Learn from your mistakes;
C. Adjust your goal;
D. Make new and more sustainable plan(s); and,
E. Commit to your new learnings.

> *Be nurturing towards the child within;
> Don't be too hard on your 'Self.'*
>
> *Accept your humanness and
> love your 'Self' unconditionally.*
>
> *Have realistic and fair expectations of yourself.
> Keep in mind that you can never be perfect.*
>
> *Source: <u>A Tool for Letting Go of Resentment and Anger:
> Short. Straightforward. Transformative.</u>*

____

____

____

____

____

____

____

____

Week 8: Your Goal and Plans for Reducing Added Sugar in Your Daily Diet

Goal(s):

Day	Plan(s)
Monday	
Tuesday	
Wednesday	
Thursday	
Friday	
Saturday	
Sunday	

Comments

Week 8 (Cont'd)

Day	Time	Deviations From Plan(s)	Calories	Comments
Monday				
Tuesday				
Wednesday				
Thursday				
Friday				
Saturday				
Sunday				

Self-Evaluation

How many times did you experience sugar cravings over the past 7 days?

____

How many times did you deviate from your original plans and give in to your temptations/cravings over the past 7 days?

____

How many calories have those deviations from your plans added to your total calorie intake for the past week?

____

Total of 3500 calories = 1 pound of body fat

Self-Reflection

*Hold yourself accountable for the deviation(s) from
your plan(s) without being self-critical.*

A. Understand what happened;
B. Learn from your mistakes;
C. Adjust your goal;
D. Make new and more sustainable plan(s); and,
E. Commit to your new learnings.

> *Love your 'Self' unconditionally.*

Hope inspires 'resolution,'
Drives 'exertion,'
Builds 'resilience,' and,
Brings 'success.'

When I earnestly hope to achieve a goal then
I will become determined to succeed.

This firm resolution will drive constructive behaviors:
I will make 'concrete plans' and exert myself
to stay committed to them.

When I stick to my plans and reap the rewards of it,
I will start believing in myself and become inspired to
stay strong and persevere in the face of setbacks.

This is how my hopes and aspirations empower me
to fulfill my vision and reach my full potential.

Source: <u>The Inner Control Is the True</u>
<u>Control Workbook, 2nd Edition</u>

*Self-awareness and self-accountability
are keys to making and maintaining
healthy lifestyle changes.*

www.ingramcontent.com/pod-product-compliance
Lightning Source LLC
Chambersburg PA
CBHW061041050726

47592CB00004B/1541